10 0526469 8

KT-149-289

OSCE: The Inside Track

OSCE: The Inside Track

Hints and tips on passing the
MRCOG Part 2 objective structured
clinical examination

Tim Draycott
Valentine Akande
Roshni Patel

University of Nottingham
at Derby Library

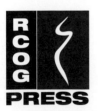

Published by the **RCOG Press** at the Royal College of Obstetricians and
Gynaecologists, 27 Sussex Place, Regent's Park, London NW1 4RG

www.rcog.org.uk

Registered charity no. 213280

First published 2005

© 2005 The Royal College of Obstetricians and Gynaecologists

No part of this publication may be reproduced, stored or transmitted in any form or
by any means, without the prior written permission of the publisher or, in the case
of reprographic reproduction, in accordance with the terms of licences issued by
the Copyright Licensing Agency in the UK [www.cla.co.uk]. Enquiries concerning
reproduction outside the terms stated here should be sent to the publisher at the UK
address printed on this page.

The use of registered names, trademarks, etc. in this publication does not imply,
even in the absence of a specific statement, that such names are exempt from the
relevant laws and regulations and therefore for general use.

While every effort has been made to ensure the accuracy of the information
contained within this publication, the publisher can give no guarantee for
information about drug dosage and application thereof contained in this book.
In every individual case the respective user must check current indications and
accuracy by consulting other pharmaceutical literature and following the guidelines
laid down by the manufacturers of specific products and the relevant authorities in
the country in which they are practising.

The rights of Tim Draycott, Valentine Akande and Roshni Patel to be identified as
Authors of this work have been asserted by them in accordance with the Copyright,
Designs and Patents Act, 1988.

ISBN 1-904752-17-9

1005264698 T

RCOG Editor: Jane Moody, assisted by Wasseema Malik
Design/typesetting by FiSH Books, London.

Printed by Latimer Trend & Co. Ltd, Estover Road, Plymouth PL6 7PL

Cover illustration by Henry Wilkinson

Contents

About the authors

Tim Draycott is a consultant in obstetrics and gynaecology at
Southmead Hospital. He started an OSCE course in the South West
region, which has been very successful: 100% of participants have
passed the OSCE examination

Valentine Akande is a consultant obstetrician and gynaecologist
and Honorary senior lecturer with the University of Bristol. He has
contributed to OSCE courses in the South West region.

Roshni Patel is a clinical academic training fellow at the University
of Bristol. She has contributed to the setting up and running of an
OSCE course in the South West region.

Top tips for approaching the OSCE

The OSCE is designed to test:

- knowledge

- the practical application of that knowledge

- its communication to a lay person.

You have the knowledge already. Now you need to demonstrate that you have the other necessary attributes. The test that many of the examiners unofficially use is: 'Would I want this person as my registrar?' 'Would I allow this doctor to treat me?'.

GENERAL INFORMATION

There are 12 stations, each of lasts 14 minutes, with 1 minute of rest between each. This is actually to let the examiners allocate marks without getting too rushed. The 15 minutes includes any reading involved, such as the patient scenario.

You are given a pencil and note pad.

The examiners are instructed not to talk to you if you finish the station early. This can be quite intimidating and you leave the station not knowing how you did. Try not to worry about this.

Of the 12 OSCE stations:

⇨ two are preparatory stations, involving, for example, critical reading of a published paper (or other document), setting priorities or compiling an audit which will be the subject of examination at the next station.

⇨ the others have a variety of formats:

- **structured viva** on a specific subject; for example, 'Tell me how you would deal with a bowel perforation ... '

- **test of technical skills**: using surgical instruments or models

- **test of communication skills**: assessing interaction with role players representing patients (or someone associated with a patient)

- history taking

- data interpretation

- emergency management

- 'bouncers', including pathology and risk management.

Read the question carefully: identify 'key words' and answer questions directly.

Remember that management includes history, examination, investigations and treatment.

This book outlines all of the different types of OSCE and a method of approaching each of them, as well as an example marking scheme for the stations so that you can see where the marks are awarded. Pass marks are based on standard setting and are therefore variable.

Read all of the examples and then practise the stations. It can be useful to practise in a group, with one person marking and one playing the candidate. It is particularly helpful to actually go though the steps and words of the station.

Approaches to individual stations

For each station, whatever the format, the examiner has a preset marking schedule with clear guidelines for what is expected of candidates. Understanding the marking schedule will make scoring easier for the OSCE itself.

GENERIC SKILLS

Part 2 examiners always emphasise that the OSCE should be approached exactly as one would at your base hospital, often with the instruction to 'be natural'. This is always a bit tricky, as most of us don't usually have an examiner in clinic. However, it is worth trying to remember that, especially when you get stuck.

At all the 'people' stations (i.e. any station with a role player) it will help your global score if you remember the following:

- introduce yourself
- use non-medical language
- make eye contact
- listen to the patient and do not interrupting
- invite questions.

Therefore, just as in the driving test where everyone exaggerates looking in the rear view mirror to make sure that the examiner has seen you do it, make sure that you emphasise these skills. Greeting the 'patient' or other person and introducing yourself, briefly explaining your role (in accordance with the instructions for that station) are normal clinical courtesies. General demeanour is important in conveying empathy, concern and attention to what the person consulting you has to say. Maintaining eye contact is one way of displaying these clinical attributes.

There may be provision for making notes during the consultation and it may be helpful to do so but preoccupation with writing rather than listening gives the wrong signals. Similarly, other displays of lack of attention, such as repeated nervous glancing at your watch, may create an even worse impression.

Counselling stations

Counselling stations are often the most intimidating. You will be asked to counsel a woman or her husband after a difficult perinatal outcome. Your approach is important. Here are a few basic rules that should help you through.

- Introduce yourself.

- Express regret at the poor outcome where appropriate.

- Ask about physical wellbeing.

- Acknowledge anger where appropriate: 'I understand that you are angry...'.

- Identify problems: 'I realise this must be difficult for you'; 'This meeting is to answer your questions'; 'Are there any questions I can help you with?'.

- Let the person talk.

- Explain in layman's language. Answer their questions directly.

- Plan for any future pregnancy: 'Some people want to know about future pregnancies. Would you like to discuss that today?'

- Offer a follow-up appointment.

- There is no absolute need to touch the patient (stroking, patting, etc.) as some candidates are prone to doing; although if you are comfortable with this and the mood takes you, you will not be marked down. Just don't feel you have to.

- Allegedly, one candidate said that she would pray for the woman. Beware of introducing religion into your consultations.

- Look at the woman and not the examiner.

- It makes sense to ask open-ended questions so that the 'patient' has to talk more and you do less. However, remember that you must do enough talking to gain marks.

TOP TIP

Have a set of prepared statements that can be applied to all distressing cases, such as:

- 'I am very sorry about your loss.'

- 'This must be a difficult time for you.'

- 'Do you have family, friends or religious support nearby?'

- 'Can I put you in touch with a counsellor?'

- 'Have you seen our bereavement midwife?'

- 'Here are some leaflets for you to read at home.'

- 'Here is our hospital number, if you want to make an appointment to talk more.'

- 'Would you like some information on support groups in the area?'

EXAMPLE TOPICS

- Counsel mother who has just lost a baby after an uncomplicated forceps delivery.

- Husband (or mother) of the above 6 weeks later, when you had no reason for the death after postmortem examination.

- A woman under your care is admitted while you are on leave for reduction in fetal movements. She is discharged home following a normal CTG. The day after she is admitted for routine induction of labour. She is diagnosed as having suffered an intrauterine death. You are seeing her (a role player) two days later.

- Six weeks later you are seeing the partner of the above patient in the clinic. All the results are normal and he is VERY angry.

- Counselling primiparous women who had been admitted at 42 weeks for induction of labour. Membranes artificially ruptured, fresh bleeding per vaginam. CTG tachy then brady. Registrar in theatre performing elective section. Decision to section made but fresh stillbirth. She was booked under your care but you were out of the country at the time. Woman (role-player) holding her head and sobbing constantly. No eye contact. Examiner observing with no input at all.

- Counselling husband (role-player) of above woman, 6 week further on. He has come alone. Wife is depressed and at her mothers. Postmortem showed baby anaemic and vasa praevia. Observing examiner.

- A woman who is anorexic and amenorrhoeic (role-player). Discuss her options as if you were in a gynaecological outpatient clinic.

- Gynaecological patient with dyspareunia and symptoms of endometriosis plus a weak family history of ovarian carcinoma. Manage as if you were in a gynaecological outpatient clinic.

Counselling stations: example 1

CANDIDATE'S INSTRUCTIONS

Mrs Harrison is a 55-year-old woman who presents with anxiety about developing ovarian cancer. A good friend of hers has recently died with the disease. Her friend had no symptoms prior to the diagnosis being made, at which point the disease was advanced. Mrs Harrison wonders whether or not there are any tests that can be performed to exclude ovarian cancer. She has seen a TV documentary. Her GP says that these tests are not locally available.

How would you establish whether there is any increased risk in her case?

Advise her about screening tests and prophylaxis.

ROLE PLAYER'S INSTRUCTIONS

You are a 55-year-old woman who works in the school meals service. You were married at age 17 and have three grown-up children, two girls and a boy. You have a sister who emigrated to Australia 30 years ago, with whom you have had very little contact, but you do know that she had been having treatment for some type of cancer last year. Your mother went to Australia to be near your sister, and she died from cancer, but you are not sure of what type – it may have been ovarian cancer.

You have been very well, you have had no operations and are not on any treatment.

A good friend of yours has recently died from ovarian cancer. She had no symptoms prior to the diagnosis being made, at which point the disease was far advanced. You are concerned about her death, but in addition, the fact that there appears to have been some deaths from cancer in your own family. You have seen a television documentary about early diagnosis of ovarian cancer but your GP says those tests are not locally available.

MARKING SCHEME

Introduction with the patient: **2 marks**

- non-medical language
- eye contact
- listens to patient/does not interrupt
- invites questions.

Candidate should enquire about family history: **2 marks**

- history of ovarian, breast, bowel cancer in mother, aunts, sisters (i.e. first-degree relatives)
- use of oral contraceptives, induction of ovulation
- number of pregnancies.

Counselling points should include: **4 marks**

- general lifetime risk of developing ovarian cancer is 1%
- most cases are sporadic
- increased risk if there is a family history, for example, a 3% lifetime risk if the patient is aged 55 years with a mother having ovarian cancer at 65 years, increasing to up to 30% if two first-degree relatives have ovarian cancer or a history of previous breast cancer, when risk is doubled
- decreased risk with increasing pregnancies and previous contraceptive pill use.

Screening tests: **4 marks**

- no current specific screening tests are available; both serum CA125 and transvaginal ultrasound are poorly predictive

- genetic tests, such as presence of *BRCA 1* gene

- presymptomatic testing is available for cancer predisposition if there is a strong family history. However, one must consider the practical and ethical difficulties, including life insurance, lack of proven benefit from intervention and implications for offspring if a carrier

- counselling in Mrs Harrison's case will depend on level of risk; depends upon type of cancer her mother and sister had.

Advice: **4 marks**

- if NO increased risk based on the history, reassure and offer no further investigation.

- if increased risk based on history as above, consider screening clinic – transvaginal ultrasound scan, serum CA125, *BRCA 1*.

- if the patient is high risk (< 30% or a *BRCA 1* gene carrier) consider oophorectomy, although this does not eliminate risk

- consider oral contraception.

Global marks   **4 marks**

TOTAL   **20 MARKS**

Counselling stations: example 2

CANDIDATE'S INSTRUCTIONS

You are the consultant obstetrician in charge of the pregnancy care of Mrs Barbara Evans who delivered a stillborn baby boy 6 weeks ago at 42 weeks of gestation, following her first pregnancy. You are now about to see her husband who has come to you in your office at his request.

You were not in the hospital at the time his wife was admitted and delivered but you did see her on the postnatal ward the following day. Mrs Barbara Evans was a 34-year-old bank clerk with an uncomplicated first pregnancy. She was due to be admitted for induction of labour for prolonged pregnancy at 42 weeks of gestation.

The day before her planned admission her husband had telephoned the labour ward for advice because Mrs Evans had noticed reduced fetal movements. After speaking to the senior midwife on duty he brought his wife into the labour ward for a cardiotocograph. The midwife had declared this to be normal (correctly) and had told Mrs Evans to go home again and return in the morning for induction of labour as previously planned. However, when Mrs Evans returned the following morning, no fetal heart sounds could be heard. Labour was induced and proceeded straightforwardly to normal delivery of a stillborn boy, who showed early signs of maceration. Postmortem examination has shown an anatomically normal male infant weighting 3.3 kg.

Your understanding is that Mrs Evans is physically well, although she is not here today, having gone away to stay with her mother in Chester. Mr Evans is angry and is demanding an explanation for the death of his son.

ROLE-PLAYER'S INSTRUCTIONS

You are Mr John Evans and your wife, Barbara, was under the care of the consultant obstetrician you are about to see with her recent first pregnancy. You are aged 32 years, a secondary school geography teacher, and your wife is 24 years old, on maternity leave from her job as a bank clerk.

Your understanding is that your wife had an uncomplicated pregnancy. She was due to be admitted for induction of labour because her pregnancy had gone overdue (2 weeks after the expected date of delivery, i.e. 42 weeks). The day before her planned admission you had telephoned the labour ward because your wife had noticed that the baby was moving less than usual. You spoke to the senior midwife on duty who told you to bring your wife up to the labour ward for monitoring, which you duly did. A monitor was put on your wife's abdomen for half an hour or so, producing a trace of the baby's heartbeat pattern. The midwife had told you that this monitoring was normal and you and your wife were told to go back home again and return to the labour ward the following morning for the planned induction.

When you and your wife arrived on the labour ward again the following morning the midwife could not hear the baby's heartbeat. A doctor came and looked at the baby with a scanning machine and told you both that the baby was dead. Your wife then had her labour induced; she had an epidural for pain relief, which was perfectly satisfactory. There were no complications with the labour and she had a normal delivery 10 hours later. The baby was a boy, whom you named James.

Your wife is physically well, but has gone away to stay with her mother in Chester. You are angry and demanding an explanation for the death of your son. You have asked for this appointment with the consultant obstetrician in order to have your questions answered and to express your dissatisfaction with your wife's care.

You are angry and quite aggressive in manner, but you should allow the candidate to introduce him or herself. Immediately after that, you start asking:

'Why did my baby die?'

'Surely they must have known there was something wrong when we came up the day before the birth?'

'Why wasn't my wife kept in hospital then?'

'Why didn't they induce her labour then?'

'I told the midwife that Barbara hadn't felt the baby moving as much as normal and all she did was put that monitor on for half an hour and tell us it was fine and we were just typical anxious first time parents, as if we were stupid'

'I am going to sue the hospital about this'.

MARKING SCHEME

Interaction with the patient: 6 marks

- Appropriate introduction.
- Sympathetic approach.
- Not responding aggressively.
- Allowing the husband to talk, not interrupting.
- Asking about his wife.
- Asking how they are coping whether counselling support is needed.
- Maintaining eye contact appropriately.

Addressing the husband's concerns: 5 marks

- Explaining fetal heart rate patterns and CTG.
- Explaining reasons for induction of labour.
- Explaining the post mortem findings in appropriate language.
- Advice for future pregnancy.

Advice: 5 marks

- Not incriminating colleagues.
- Not becoming agitated by intention to sue.
- Explaining access to complaints procedure.
- Offering to meet again with his wife and the carer.
- Offering to discuss management for a future pregnancy.

Global marks 4 marks

TOTAL 20 MARKS

Counselling stations: example 3

CANDIDATE'S INSTRUCTIONS

The woman you are about to see is attending the hospital for a routine antenatal visit at 35 weeks of gestation. Before you go to see her, the midwife speaks to you outside the room. She is concerned about the woman, who she says is complaining of rather vague symptoms of headache and generalised aches and pains. She is not sleeping and appears to have multiple bruising on her body that she is reluctant to explain.

You have 15 minutes to see, and advise the patient as you feel necessary based on the outcome of your consultation.

ROLE PLAYER'S INSTRUCTIONS

You are 24 years old, this is your first pregnancy and you have reached 35 weeks of gestation.

This pregnancy was unplanned. You booked at the maternity hospital at 12 weeks of gestation. You were last seen in the hospital at 18 weeks. You are sharing antenatal care with GP but have not attended very often. There have been no obstetric complications to date but you have been having domestic problems with your partner.

You and your partner, Billy, were married last year and you got pregnant soon after. Billy works as an estate agent. Recently, he claims to have been under a lot of pressure at work and has been spending more time than usual away from home. You recently moved to his area and have no family or friends who live nearby.

Soon after you were married he began to beat you physically. This has continued throughout your pregnancy and you no longer feel safe at home. He returned home late last night, offering no explanation of where he had been. You argued and eventually he beat you viciously. This has happened before on about five occasions.

You now feel you need help but don't know where to turn.

You are now attending the antenatal clinic in the hospital for the first time since early pregnancy (you saw the GP). The midwife has noticed the bruising and you also mentioned you have had problems with vague headaches, generalised pains and poor sleeping. She has gone to get the doctor.

The doctor believes this is a routine visit but should be suspicious about the bruising, as the midwife has specifically mentioned it to him or her. If he or she enquires about the bruising you should open up and discuss he true situation. If, after a few minutes, the doctor makes no effort to discuss the bruising, you should initiate discussion about your domestic situation.

Mention:

- unable to cope with the violence
- no longer feel safe at home
- you feel it's your fault and you feel powerless
- frightened of officialdom/agencies
- fearful of repercussions of disclosure.

MARKING SCHEME

Introduction: 4 marks

- Language
- Contact
- Personal details
- Current pregnancy
- Social/personal history

Enquires about bruising: 5 marks

- Sympathetic about bruising
- Ability to listen
- Relevance of direct questions
- Nonjudgmental
- Emotional support
- Confidentiality (except mental health order
  and child protection procedures).

Relevance of advice: 5 marks

- Contact numbers
- Legal options
- Help for perpetrators
- Remove from at risk situation
- Friends or relatives
- Social worker
- Woman's Aid help line
- Temporary accommodation

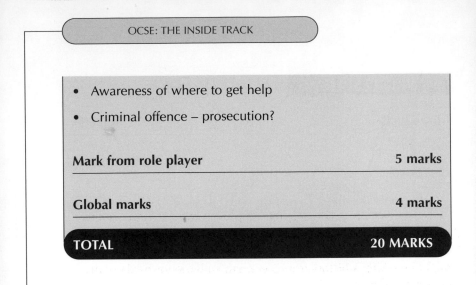

- Awareness of where to get help

- Criminal offence – prosecution?

Mark from role player	**5 marks**
Global marks	**4 marks**
TOTAL	**20 MARKS**

History-taking stations

These stations are potentially the simplest, although marks in the examinations are often surprisingly low. They lend themselves well to the 'think you're in clinic' approach to OSCE. A typical station might be taking a history from a woman with menorrhagia with a GP's referral letter.

Work through a history in the standard way:

- presenting complaint

- history of the complaint, including previous treatment

- previous medical history (the 'patient' will usually have been briefed to have had a deep vein thrombosis while taking the pill or something similar for you to find)

- social history, such as who might be at home to help

- quality-of-life assessment (for example, social restrictions)

- obstetric history for the index pregnancy can usefully be divided into trimesters:
  - first trimester, including booking (drugs, smoking and social support) and threatened miscarriage
  - second trimester: anomaly scan
  - third trimester: whatever since.

- previous obstetric history.

The examiner may provide details of any examination required. Allow time to discuss treatment options at the end; only half the marks are allocated to the history alone.

Remember to think of a differential diagnosis and explain this to the 'patient' with a management plan. Start with the simplest and most conservative treatment options. Let her ask questions (she will have been briefed for this).

As always, there are generic marks available – see page 3.

If a surgical treatment is being considered then make an assessment of the anaesthetic fitness of the patient as well as making a note of possible complications.

TOP TIP

General questions at the end may pick up missed information:

- 'Is there anything else that you are worried about?'
- 'Has anything happened recently which has caused you concern?'
- 'Are you happy with this plan?'

EXAMPLE TOPICS

28/40 gestation pregnant woman who is small for dates. Take the history from a patient with intrauterine growth restriction and reduction of fetal movements. Given the results of the physical examination from the examiner. Explain the possible options to the woman.

35/40 gestation pregnant women with bruising. Expected to discover history of domestic violence and offer constructive advice.

Midwife asks you to see someone she is concerned about. No notes available. Take history. You are given the results of the examination (role-player with examiner observing).

Take the history from a woman with incontinence (role-player).
You are then given the results of the physical examination from the
examiner. Explain to the woman her possible options.

30-year-old woman referred by her GP with 1-year history of
discharge (role-player). Manage as if you were in a gynaecological
outpatient clinic. At end of history, you are given a piece of paper
with the findings of the examination and the results of an
ultrasound scan, which were normal. Then discuss management
plan. Examiner observing.

MARKING SCHEME

History taking: menorrhagia

Introduction: 2 marks

- eye contact

- listens to patient/does not interrupt

- invites questions.

Takes full history: 3 marks

- enquires about other treatments tried so far: tranexamic acid,
  mefanamic acid, progestogen, levonorgestrel-releasing
  intrauterine system

- asks about relationship/stability, premenstrual symptoms.

Management: 6 marks

- conservative management to avoid hysterectomy

- endometrial ablation – either laser or resection, thermal

- if surgery contemplated, conserves ovaries

- discusses types of hysterectomy and potential difficulties
- hysterectomy – subtotal versus total.

Risk of surgery: **5 marks**

- obesity
- anaesthesia
- bladder injury or trauma
- bowel injury due to adhesions
- deep vein thrombosis/pulmonary embolism
- chest infections and others
- haemorrhage
- electrolyte imbalance (hyponatraemia).

Global marks   **4 marks**

TOTAL   **20 MARKS**

Critical appraisal stations

This station involves appraisal of a leaflet, journal article, internet print-out or even possibly an advertisement. There will be a preparatory station and you will be given a pencil and paper to make notes about the text.

LEAFLET

The examiners are looking for discussion of the following general categories:

- Is the content comprehensive and accurate? You need to demonstrate a working knowledge of the subject of the leaflet or article.

- Is the language of the leaflet appropriate for a layperson? Are the leaflets translated into other languages as well as English?

- Consider the layout and presentation – is it easy to follow?

- Is there sufficient follow-up information?

TOP TIP

Make a mental checklist of things you need to discuss. For example:

- When was the leaflet written?
- Who was it written by?
- Is there a contact point for further enquiries?
- Is it available in other languages than English?
- Is it in plain, clear English?
- Are any diagrams explained?
- Is a glossary included?

JOURNAL ARTICLE

This short book cannot teach the finer points of critical appraisal. It is a skill that we should all learn and there are many books and web resources that cover it in detail. However, there are some basics that should be covered.

1. Is there a clearly stated objective?

Ask why the study is being performed. The objectives should be clearly stated; for example, 'to determine whether the incidence of wound infections is reduced by the preoperative administration of co-amoxiclav' is a clearly stated specific objective, as opposed to a vague desire 'to assess the value of prophylactic antibiotics in surgery'.

2. Is the study design appropriate to the objective?

Where an intervention, such as a new drug, is being evaluated, the gold standard is the prospective randomised controlled trial. This should allow comparison between the new treatment and the older treatment, or the new treatment versus no treatment at all (or placebo). When assessing the aetiology of a condition, patients with the condition can be compared with people without the disease but similar in all other respects (for example, age, social class, ethnicity, parity).

3. **Has the study been performed on a sample representative of the population being studied?**

    This would include the sample size and the sampling method. Sample size should have been decided prior to the study using a power calculation, taking into account the expected impact of the intervention. Were there clearly defined criteria for patient inclusion and exclusion? What was done about patients who were invited to join the study but refused?

4. **Is there a suitable control group? Is the control group comparable to the treatment group?**

    Subjects should be randomised to treatment and control groups. Randomisation should ensure that the two groups are similar with regard to known confounding factors.

5. **Have the outcome measures been stated clearly?**

    It is important to know what measures were used to assess the effect of the intervention, such as days in hospital, caesarean section rates or perinatal mortality. In some circumstances, there are questions relating to the validity and reproducibility of outcome measures, such as results of hormonal assays or subjective pain scores.

6. **Are we being shown the whole picture?**

    In most studies there is bound to be a certain number of patients who do not complete the study, for one reason or another. Do the authors supply their details? Is the amount of missing data sufficient to detract from the overall validity of the conclusions?

7. **Are there factors that might have distorted the results?**

   Are there differences between the control and treatment groups that might impact on the outcome? Care should be taken when comparing noncontemporaneous groups because there may have been changes over time that cannot be controlled for.

8. **Have the data been analysed by appropriate statistical methods?**

   Statistical method selection is vitally important. The majority of studies do not need esoteric or highly complicated statistical manoeuvres to make their point (beware the three-tailed James-Akande test with the Marquis de Sade correction factor for $n = 1$ studies).

TOP TIP

Get involved in a department journal club. Better to embarrass oneself in front of the department and learn from it, rather than when Part 2 is at stake.

EXAMPLE TOPICS

- Patient information sheet review.

- You are given the RCOG information leaflet on hysterectomy. You have 15 minutes to read it and then appraise it with the examiner.

- You are given a leaflet prepared by RCOG for patients, about endometriosis. Assess, criticise and suggest improvements. Discuss aforementioned leaflet with examiner.

Critical appraisal stations: example

CANDIDATE'S INFORMATION (PREPARATORY STATION)

Read the pamphlet entitled *Cervical Smears*. You may write (make notes) on the copy of the pamphlet you are reading and must take it with you to the next station.

At the next station you will be asked to appraise the pamphlet and discuss its value and limitations with the examiner (15 minutes).

You will be awarded marks for your ability to critically appraise the pamphlet.

You must leave the pamphlet with the examiner.

CANDIDATE'S INSTRUCTIONS

Please read the pamphlet on *Cervical Smears*. Comment on its strength and weakness.

EXAMINER'S INFORMATION

As an examiner you will need to read the information pamphlet, *Cervical Smears*.

Your candidate has had 15 minutes at the previous station to read the pamphlet, to consider its value and limitations and to prepare him or herself for questions you are going to ask.

Ask the candidate to tell you the value and the limitations of the pamphlet and any other comments/observations he or she might have.

EXAMINER'S NOTES

- Understates a little, evolution from CIN to cancer, gives false sense of security.

- Does not explain the difference between treatment and observation for CIN1.

- There should be more emphasis to investigating women who never had a smear.

- Practice in 1980 should be omitted.

- Preferably avoid treatment during menses.

- Management in pregnancy not mentioned.

- Not enough on 'inadequate smear' report.

- If symptoms develop, should be referred to a gynaecologist, rather than have smear testing done.

- Advice after colposcopy – driving, work, sexual intercourse.

- Follow up important not sufficient detailed or emphasised.

- Meaning of medical terms CIN – not in outlining of the neck of the womb. Dyskaryosis should be explained in lay person's terms.

Please collect pamphlet from the candidate.

MARKING SCHEME

Candidates should be rated for the following abilities:

Demonstrates clear understanding of the subject matter of the pamphlet.	4 marks
Identifies the generally comprehensive nature but recognises that there are several important deficiencies.	4 marks
Pinpoints deficiencies without leading questions. If lead required, loses mark.	4 marks
Is able to make an overall evaluation of the content of the pamphlet.	4 marks
Global marks	4 marks
TOTAL	**20 MARKS**

Audit stations

The most common mistake is to assume that you need to research the subject, rather than audit it; for example, trying to demonstrate that Foley catheters are useful for 24 hours after caesarean section, rather than auditing whether hospital staff are complying with the hospital protocol, which states that they should have a catheter in place for 24 hours after a caesarean section. Remember: research sets standards and audit measures how closely we are complying with those standards.

Most commonly, there will be a preparatory station where you will be given 15 minutes to plan your audit. The audit topic will be described and you are expected to detail all the steps of the audit cycle.

The audit cycle is composed of the following steps:

1. Define a standard, e.g. 100% compliance with protocol.

2. Measure compliance to that standard:
    prospective/retrospective review of data and sample size.

3. Analyse data, including 'missing data'.

4. Present results.

5. Identify changes that would help.

6. Re-audit after changes.

TOP TIP

Prepare an outline of how the ideal audit should be conducted. This should contain about ten points and should complete the audit cycle. Any audit with which you are faced can then be easily adapted to fit and top marks should be forthcoming. Remember to use a multi-professional approach and include points on cost evaluation and involving mangers.

EXAMPLE TOPICS

■ Review a hospital's current practice in a district audit unit.

■ Your unit has a detailed protocol for the management of intrauterine growth restriction. You are asked to audit how the protocol is adhered to in the unit.

■ Discuss the design of an audit protocol with an examiner. It investigated the level of adherence to a protocol for the management of post dates pregnancy in a district audit unit. General discussion of audit, e.g. prospective/retrospective, standards, targets. What to do with results. How to follow up, etc.

MARKING SCHEME

Audit

Examiner will award marks for the following:

- **Describing the key components of an audit:**   **10 marks**

- **Feeding the results back to the department:**   **4 marks**

- **Considering whether any changes are required in the department to improve compliance:**   **4 marks**

- **Considering whether the protocol needs modification, e.g. in the light of any recent Department of Health/RCOG guidelines, etc:**   **4 marks**

- **Date for re-audit:**   **4 marks**

Global marks   **4 marks**

TOTAL   **20 MARKS**

Audit stations: example

This is a station with a preparatory station.

CANDIDATE'S INFORMATION

In a district general hospital, five consultants agree a new policy that all women undergoing a hysterectomy should be catheterised with a No. 12 Foley catheter, which will routinely be removed 48 hours postoperatively. This agreement was based on the evidence that intermittent catheterisation appears to increase the rate of urinary infection compared with an indwelling catheter. Conduct an audit as to whether the practice in their unit accords with the protocol.

EXAMINER'S INSTRUCTIONS

The candidate needs to cover the five areas of discussion detailed in the marking scheme and may be prompted if he or she doe not mention them spontaneously. Deduct marks for prompting.

MARKING SCHEME

Describe the key components of an audit: **8 marks**

- Which patients should have been managed by this protocol in the given time period
- Would a x% sample be sufficient
- Determine method of establishing whether the protocol was followed for each patient
- Ascertain the outcome
- Analyse data including quantifying missing data
- Identifying why the protocol was not followed in some areas.

Feed results back to departmental staff: **3 marks**

- Sensitively
- Consider confidentiality
- What reactions might be expected.

Consider if organisational changes are needed to facilitate improve compliance: **3 marks**

- Resource implications
- How to achieve consistent implementation.

Consider if any element of protocol requires modification: **1 mark**

- Recent research data/College guidelines
- Has there been criticism + protocol by user group.

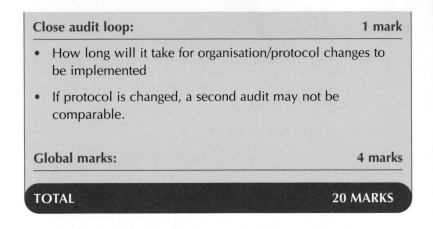

Close audit loop: 1 mark

- How long will it take for organisation/protocol changes to be implemented

- If protocol is changed, a second audit may not be comparable.

Global marks: 4 marks

TOTAL 20 MARKS

Obstetric prioritisation stations

This is a key station and usually comprises a labour ward board. You will have 15 minutes to prepare for this station. You will be provided with relevant details of each woman and also be told about the staff available and their level of experience.

You will be expected to list all the tasks required on the labour ward. The examiner is looking for your ability to prioritise and order these tasks. He or she will want you to consider both fetal and maternal wellbeing.

Read the information provided in detail. Work through one patient at a time so that you do not miss important facts. There is enough time to do this. Keep 'clinical priorities' in mind all the way through.

It is difficult to achieve a precise order. Start by trying to group the cases into three categories: high, medium and low. High and low tend to be the clearest, the remainder slot into the middle order. Having done this, it will be easier to assign a more defined order within each group. There will be some flexibility in ordering the cases, especially in the middle ranking. It is more important that you are able to justify your choice of order.

Write notes on the information sheet to save time, rather than copying the details to your note pad.

Let the examiner know how you will be approaching this problem: 'I will order the cases into high, medium and low priority. I will identify the individual problems of each woman and their management. I will implement...'. This helps to set the scene.

TOP TIP

Do not fall into obvious gaffes, such as saying that an IVF pregnancy is a precious pregnancy or that Lady X needs urgent review on account of her title.

Obstetric prioritisation stations: example

CANDIDATE'S INSTRUCTIONS

You are the registrar on call for the delivery unit. You have just arrived for the handover at 08.30. Attached you will find a brief resume of the ten women on the delivery suite, as shown on the board. The staff available today are:

- an obstetric SHO in her fourth month of GP training

- a third-year specialist anaesthetic registrar

- the consultant on call is in his gynaecology clinic and is not keen on being disturbed unless absolutely necessary

- six midwives: SW is in charge; SW, CK and MC can suture episiotomies; DB, SW and PV can insert an intravenous line.

Read the board carefully. You have 15 minutes to decide what tasks need to be done, in which order they should be done and who should be allocated to each task.

At the next station you will meet the examiner, with whom you will discuss your decisions and your reasoning.

You will be awarded marks for your ability to manage the delivery suite.

EXAMINER'S INSTRUCTIONS

The candidate has 15 minutes to explain to you the following:

- the tasks which need doing on delivery suite.

- the order in which the candidate would do them and which staff he or she would allocate to each.

MARKING SCHEME

Tasks required: **10 marks**

Room 1. Review blood pressure, urine output, proteinuria, pain relief, blood loss, general condition postoperatively, drug regimen.

Room 2. Assess progress. Why not delivered?

Room 3. Needs discussion of abdominal versus vaginal delivery; full blood count and group in case of lower segment caesarean section.

Room 4. Needs assessment and more information.

Room 5. Need to check progress and deliver.

Room 6. Need to check CTG and progress. Confirm blood sent for full blood count and group and save.

Room 7. Check consent and that blood has been sent for full blood count, group and save.

Room 8. Needs suturing.

Room 9. No action required.

Room 10. Assess if in labour. Check fetal and maternal wellbeing. Check neonatal cots. Decide mode of delivery.

Priority of tasks and staff allocation: **10 marks**

- Urgent review by registrar in rooms 6, 2 and 5.
- Semi-urgent review by registrar in rooms 3 and 10.
- SHO to assess room 4.
- Routine review in room 1, SHO and anaesthetist.
- Non-urgent review in room 7.
- Midwife to suture in room 8.
- No need for doctor to see room 9.

TOTAL   **20 MARKS**

Room	Name	Para	Gestation (weeks)	Liquor	Epidural	Syntocinon	Comments	MW
1	Owusu	1+1	32	–	Yes	Yes	LSCS at 0100 (PET) EBL 800 ml baby on SCBU	SW
2	Evans	2+0	T+9	Meconium	Yes	No	7cm at 0300 Domino	Com/MW
3	Arnold	0+0	39	Intact	No	No	Undiagnosed breech Spontaneous labour; 4 cm at 0730 Breech at spines	SW
4	McDonald	0+0	28				Dr to see Abdominal pain CTG normal	MC
5	Winston	0+0	41	Meconium	Yes	No	Fully dilated at 0700	VM
6	Khan	1+0 LSCS	T+2	Clear	No	No	Trial of scar. ARM at 0300 FBS at 0600 pH 7.29 6 cm at 0600	DB
7	Jenkins	2+0	38	Intact	No	No	Routine admission for LSCS	VM
8	Birch	0+0	39				Delivered, awaiting suturing	PL
9	Nash	2+0	T+6	Intact	No	No	Spontaneous labour; 3cm at 0650	MC
10	Collins	0+2	33	1	No	No	Twins, contracting. Ceph/ceph IVF pregnancy	PL

OBSTETRIC PRIORITISATION

Gynaecology prioritisation stations

This usually comprises a consultant's gynaecology waiting list (see example table). You will be given 15 minutes to prepare for this station. There will usually be ten cases, each of which you will have to prioritise. You will be asked to discuss each case briefly. You will be provided with relevant details of each woman and also be told about the staff available and their level of experience.

This station requires a slightly different approach to the obstetric prioritisation station and it is advisable to discuss each case in turn. You will be expected to identify clearly the appropriate operative investigation or treatment for each case (for example, laparoscopy, laparotomy, LLETZ, vaginal hysterectomy, myomectomy). You should be able to justify your decision based on the specific details given for the patient.

The examiner will also want you to indicate the appropriate venue each procedure; e.g. inpatient, day case or possibly outpatient (for example, hysteroscopy).

You will be required to identify special circumstances that require additional attention and how you will deal with them, such as social difficulties, Jehovah's Witnesses, previous abdominal surgery, preoperative comorbidities such as anaemia, obesity or immunocompromisation. You will need to be able to discuss the use of anaesthetic preoperative assessment for such cases. In complicated cases, you should indicate that it would be necessary for a consultant or other specialist, such as a general surgeon, to be present.

The examiner will also be assessing your ability to prioritise these cases, according to three categories: urgent, soon or routine/in turn. These should be according to clinical priority, i.e. potential malignancy, then morbidity, in order.

Read the information provided in detail. Work through one patient at a time so that you do not miss important facts. There is enough time to do this.

Use the table given to prompt you for each case: go through each column heading for each operation. Even if you are personally very experienced and competent, in difficult cases, make it clear that a consultant must be present for the operation as this is what is expected at pre-MRCOG level. In ambiguous cases, be flexible in your approach. For example, an operation might be successfully performed laparoscopically but if this proves impossible a laparotomy might be necessary. The operative arrangements should reflect this, so it may be best to admit her as an inpatient on the understanding that if a laparotomy proves unnecessary she might go home on the same day. In patients with previous medical difficulties, the candidate would be expected to discuss the preoperative treatment, such as correction of the anaemia and the prerequisite of a normal blood count prior to surgery. Do not say that very elderly patients are not a priority because of their age alone.

TOP TIP

Think about what happens in real, everyday practice and not what would happen in private practice.

Gynaecology prioritisation stations: example

CANDIDATE'S INSTRUCTIONS

You are asked to go through a consultant's gynaecology waiting list and advise the waiting list manager on:

1.   Appropriate procedure(s) (operation and others).

2.   Venue of proposed treatment.

3.   Special needs.

4.   Priority assignment.

Please describe your action and offer explanation wherever appropriate.

You will be awarded marks for your ability to manage and prioritise the cases, with reasoning for your actions.

EXAMINER'S INSTRUCTIONS

Discuss each case briefly. As long as there is consistency and safety, score according to the confidence of the candidate's priority setting.

Extra notes

AB: It should be clear that a consultant must be present for this operation.

KR: This operation might be successfully performed laparoscopically but if this proves impossible a laparotomy may be necessary. The operative arrangements should reflect this, so it may be best to admit the woman as an inpatient on the understanding that, if a laparotomy proves unnecessary, she might go home on the same day. The special needs arrangement for the care of her invalid child would have to reflect the 'worst case' scenario.

QT: The operation could include either total abdominal hysterectomy or subtotal hysterectomy (not myomectomy). The candidate should discuss the preoperative treatment of the anaemia and the prerequisite of a normal blood count prior to surgery. Although oral iron may be sufficient, the discussion should also include hormonal ovarian suppression if this fails. The special operation consent form is best completed prior to admission.

TN: The use of anaesthetic preoperative assessment should be discussed.

TL: This patient is best admitted as an inpatient because of the possibility of bowel damage during laparoscopy. She should be warned of this risk.

MARKING SCHEME

A. Logical action (operation and others):	8 marks
B. Venue of proposed treatment:	3 marks
C. Special needs:	3 marks
D. Priority assignment:	6 marks
TOTAL	**20 MARKS**

CANDIDATE'S INFORMATION: WAITING LIST FOR OPERATIONS

Name	Age (years)	Details	Operation and logical action	Venue	Special needs	Priority
JA	28	Deep dyspareunia, menorrhagia, ovarian cyst (8 cm) Scan suggests benign cyst				
AB	42	Large pelvic mass Likely ovarian cyst Serum CA125 = 45 iu/ml				
JF	18	Recent abnormal smear Cervical biopsy CIN3 Request treatment under GA				
PH	30	P3+1; recent termination of pregnancy				
		History of subacute bacterial endocarditis and deep vein thrombosis Wishes laparoscopic sterilisation				
PR	18	Primary amenorrhoea/cyclical pain Ultrasound shows distended vagina				
KR	32	P5+0; Missing IUCD (IUCD in abdominal cavity) Caring for invalid child				
QT	44	Fibroid uterus, menorrhagia Haemoglobin 8.1 Jehovah's Witness				
TN	82	Recent angina (failed pessary) Procidentia Lives alone, incontinent				
TL	28	Laparoscopy for pain, previous laparotomy (twice)				
JB	22	Secondary subfertility for 3 years Previous ectopic pregnancy				

Equipment stations

You will be presented with an instrument or piece of equipment in common use in gynaecological practice. There is only a limited number of items that you can be shown and it would seem sensible to check the following: hysteroscope, laparoscope, cystoscope, diathermy instruments.

For each instrument you will need to:

- describe the instrument, including assembly, and, where appropriate, angle of scope, etc.

- list and discuss indications for the use of the instrument or equipment

- list and discuss contraindications to use of the instrument or equipment

- potential complications and alternative options.

If you really do not recognise something, just describe it. Do not be thrown by making a mistake. For example, if you identify a cystoscope as a laparoscope the examiner will correct you and then you are back on track, having probably lost only minimal marks.

Pick up the instrument. If asked to, assemble the parts – with care, as rough and inappropriate handling of instruments does not give a good impression.

TOP TIP

Check out the finer points of diathermy: monopolar and bipolar. Learn to distinguish between single-use (disposable) and multiple-use instruments.

EXAMPLE TOPICS

- Put together a hysteroscope and discuss its use.

- There is a laparoscope on the table. You are asked to assemble it and to describe its use.

- Assemble a cystoscope and then talk through a cystoscopy.

Equipment stations: example

CANDIDATE'S INSTRUCTIONS

The examiner will show you some instruments and will ask you questions about them.

You will be marked on your ability to demonstrate your familiarity with the instruments, their correct use and limitations.

EXAMINER'S INSTRUCTIONS

You have in front of you a hysteroscope with accessories. Ask the candidate:

- What type of hysteroscope? Rigid, any other type?

- Describe the instrument and enumerate the accessories that are required.

- Describe the indications for using hysteroscope, both for diagnostic and therapeutic purposes.

- What are the contraindications to the use of hysteroscope?

- What complications may arise following a diagnostic or therapeutic hysteroscopy?

- Alternative investigations for dysfunctional uterine bleeding (endometrial sampling, transvaginal sonography, saline distension sonography); how do they compare with hysteroscopy?

MARKING SCHEME

A. Knowledge of the instruments: 3 marks

- Correct description of accessories and instruments.

B. Indications for use of hysteroscopy as an inpatient/outpatient for diagnostic and therapeutic purposes: 4 marks

- Bleeding conditions
- Menorrhagia, intermenstrual bleeding, post menopausal bleeding
- Suspected cancer or hyperplasia of the endometrium
- Recurrent miscarriage
- Infertility
- Therapeutic – resection/ablation, fibroid, septa.

C. Contraindications: 3 marks

- Suspected pregnancy
- Haemorrhagic disorders, anticoagulation
- Infection.

D. Complications: 3 marks

- Ascending infection
- Perforation
- Haemorrhage
- Hyponatraemia
- Cervical stenosis, synechiae.

E. Alternative to hysteroscopy: 3 marks

- Endometrial sampling
- Transvaginal ultrasound sonography
- Saline distension sonography.

Global marks 4 marks

TOTAL **20 MARKS**

Data or procedure stations

You will be presented with a specific procedure or data commonly seen in gynaecological practice. This is another of the 'just as if you were doing it' situations. They usually tend to cover surgical operations or data interpretation. There is no patient and the examiner will discuss the case with you.

PROCEDURE

In the case of an operation or procedure, think chronologically and include all steps. Be systematic and imagine yourself in the real-life situation. Use specific names, such as cefuroxime and metronidazole rather than just 'antibiotics'. As you describe the procedure chronologically, attempt to justify concisely each step. It probably would be sensible to practise discussing common surgical operations, particularly vaginal hysterectomy.

The following would be a sensible system for approaching an operative question:

- preoperative preparation, including thromboprophylaxis and antibiotics
- peroperative preparation, including assessment and preparation of the patient, positioning and catheterisation
- detailed operative procedure
- postoperative course.

EXAMPLE TOPICS

■ Discuss the steps required to perform a caesarean section for a transverse lie at term.

■ Lower segment caesarean section: woman with placenta praevia; discuss the operative procedure and potential complications.

■ Primiparous woman on labour ward stuck at 8 cm despite 6 hours of oxytocin. No epidural. CTG fine. Head deeply engaged. Decision been made to perform caesarean section. You are walking to theatre with your consultant (examiner), who is going to assist you. Take him through the management of the patient, including talking to the patient about the section. Also take him through the section.

■ You are in labour ward with your consultant (the examiner). A woman, para 3, in labour at 3 cm, has transverse lie and suboptimal CTG. She will undergo caesarean section. You have to explain and discus with the consultant (examiner) all the different steps (i.e. choice of incision, anaesthetic etc.).

■ A woman has a clear history of polycystic ovaries (irregular light periods, greasy skin, recent and gradual increase of weight). You are presented with her blood results (all normal) and a scan report showing a typical picture of polycystic ovaries. You have to explain to the examiner (as if he or she were the patient) the condition, the options for treatment and the possible future implications.

■ Girl in her 20s (played by examiner) with irregular periods after stopping pill, referred by her GP. Ultrasound scan arranged and referred. Also noticed dry skin and weight gain. Blood results given: luteinising hormone – 5.8; follicle-stimulating hormone – 4.5; thyroid-stimulating hormone – 1.1; prolactin – 1874; testosterone – 1.3; oestradiol 125 pmol. Ultrasound showed normal-sized uterus with normal endometrial thickening. Ovaries 1.2 × 2.1 × 1.4 cm. Two cysts less than 10 mm noted in right ovary. Discuss as in clinic.

DATA

There are a number of data sessions, commonly covering data relating to endocrinology, such as: polycystic ovary syndrome (high luteinising hormone/follicle-stimulating hormone ratio), raised prolactin levels and hypothyroidism or infertility data such as semen analysis.

Indicate which results are abnormal. Make a differential diagnosis using the data available. Think about the clinical context in which the data are presented and how this would influence management of the patient.

Explain the results in layman's terms.

You should be able to discuss management options, including possible further investigations and potential treatment options.

TOP TIP

Revise some endocrinology and infertility data. Be conversant with ultrasound scans and the biochemical diagnosis of PCOS.

Data stations: example 1

CANDIDATE INSTRUCTIONS

You are a doctor in a colposcopy clinic. Miss Spain is a 26-year-old nulliparous woman who has been referred after an abnormal routine smear. Please read the cytology report below and explain it to Miss Spain (the examiner) with details of any management plan.

> **St. Elsewhere's Hospital, Department of Cytopathology.**
> **Cytology report**
> **Routine cervical smear – moderate dyskaryosis.**

EXAMINER'S INSTRUCTIONS

The candidate is expected to be able to explain and advise after an abnormal smear result – moderate dyskaryosis. The candidate is a doctor in a colposcopy clinic. Miss Spain is a 26-year-old nulliparous woman who has been referred after a routine smear which was reported as moderate dyskaryosis. You are Miss Spain. Please give the candidate the cytology report and ask him or her to explain it to you and thereafter the relevant management. After he or she has explained the result and discussed the options of colposcopy and biopsy, give the candidate the histology report and ask him or her to explain it and the subsequent management.

> **St. Elsewhere's Hospital, Department of Histology**
> **Cervical biopsy**
> **CIN III**

MARKING SCHEME

Manner with the patient:	2 marks
Explanation of dyskaryosis:	2 marks
Reassurance that it is not malignant:	2 marks
Referral for colposcopy:	2 marks
Description of colposcopy:	2 marks
Would perform loop excision:	2 marks
Explanation of procedure:	2 marks
Potential risks:	2 marks
Significance of CIN II:	2 marks
Follow up:	2 marks
TOTAL	**20 MARKS**

Data stations: example 2

CANDIDATE'S INSTRUCTIONS

You are the registrar in the Subfertility Clinic. A young couple has returned for the results of the preliminary investigations you ordered. They have a 2-year history of primary subfertility. All the results for the female partner are normal.

shown below. Please could you take a history and explain the significance of the results and any management options. He is apparently healthy.

The examiner is the male partner.

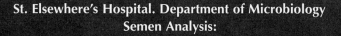

St. Elsewhere's Hospital. Department of Microbiology
Semen Analysis:

Sperm count: 5 million per ml
Motility: 30%
Abnormal forms: 60%
Leucocytes: few

EXAMINER'S INSTRUCTIONS

The candidate is expected to be able to manage an abnormal semen analysis appropriately. A young couple has returned for the results of the preliminary investigations he has ordered. They have a 2-year history of primary subfertility. All the results for the female partner are normal. The report of the male partner's semen analysis are given. Ask the candidate to take a history, explain the significance of the results and any management options.

You play the role of the male partner.

MARKING SCHEME

Checking that patient had abstained prior to producing
sample and not on any treatment or had illness in last
6–8 weeks: 1 mark

Explanation of semen analysis to include: 5 marks

- significant oligospermia

- low motility

- low normal forms

Explaining that results may vary considerably from week to
week therefore need to repeat although, as all parameters
abnormal, likely will require assisted conception   1 mark

Treatment options (briefly):   7 marks

- IVF

- ICSI

- option of donor insemination (if assisted conception
  unacceptable)

- still small chance of spontaneous conception

Global marks: 4 marks

TOTAL   20 MARKS

Procedure stations: example

CANDIDATE INSTRUCTIONS

Please explain to the examiner how you would conduct a vaginal hysterectomy, including the pre- and postoperative management.

EXAMINER'S INSTRUCTIONS

The candidate is expected to be able to talk through the techniques required for a vaginal hysterectomy, including the pre- and postoperative management. Where the candidate deviates from the marking scheme, marks should be awarded if there is an appropriate justification.

MARKING SCHEME

Preoperative: **2 marks**

- antibiotics
- thromboembolic deterrent stockings
- heparin/clexane

Operative preparation: **5 marks**

- anaesthesia
- positioning
- prep
- bimanual assessment
- ± catheterise (justify choice)
- ± infiltration (justify choice)

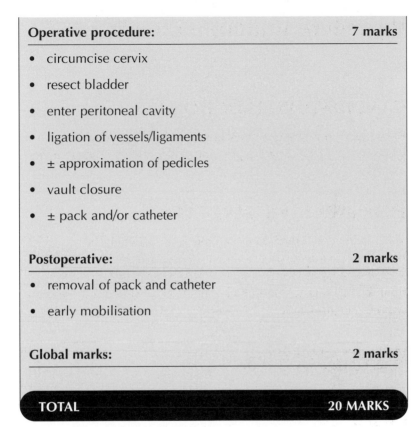

Operative procedure: 7 marks

- circumcise cervix
- resect bladder
- enter peritoneal cavity
- ligation of vessels/ligaments
- ± approximation of pedicles
- vault closure
- ± pack and/or catheter

Postoperative: 2 marks

- removal of pack and catheter
- early mobilisation

Global marks: 2 marks

TOTAL **20 MARKS**

Emergency stations

In general, there are three main areas to consider in any kind of emergency:

- get appropriate help
- general measures
- specific measures.

Imagine that you are talking to your SHO or an eager medical student, i.e. someone you feel confident enough to give instructions to.

Always start with the A B C of resuscitation in any case of haemorrhage or collapse.

Be familiar with the drugs or fluids you would use and in what quantity you would use them.

Make sure you involve other specialists, as this was one of the recommendations in the last Confidential Enquiry into Maternal Deaths in the United Kingdom.

Do not skimp on investigations – money is no object here!

TOP TIP

The icing on the cake, if you say everything you can, includes discussion of thorough note keeping, completing an incident form and debriefing (of staff and patient).

EXAMPLE TOPIC

- You perforate a uterus during an evacuation of the retained products of conception. What would you do?

Emergency stations: example 1

CANDIDATE INSTRUCTIONS

You have 15 minutes to review the scenario below and answer the questions.

You are a registrar performing a laparotomy for an ovarian cyst. There are adhesions and when you divide the adhesions, you notice faeces. The woman has a previous history of appendicectomy. Your consultant is performing a Wertheim's hysterectomy and is half way through.

1. What do you do?

2. What should you do while you are waiting?

3. Help arrives in the form of a surgical consultant. He finds a 2 cm hole in the sigmoid colon: what is he likely to do?

   Unfortunately, there is no ovarian cyst, merely a collection of intraperitoneal fluid. The ovaries are adherent to the pelvic sidewall. No further dissection was attempted.

4. Describe any measures you would take before closing the abdomen and technique for closure.

5. How would you explain the operation to the patient and her relatives postoperatively?

EXAMINER'S INSTRUCTIONS

The candidate has 15 minutes to review a clinical scenario of an inadvertent bowel injury. You should look for safe, acceptable practice and risk management principles.

MARKING SCHEME

What do you do?   **3 marks**

- Recognised problem – bowel perforation
- Stop operation
- Contact consultant
- Call senior surgical assistant.

What would you do while you are waiting?   **3 marks**

- Antibiotics
- Nasogastric tube·
- Prevent spread of faeces – local packing.

What is the surgical consultant likely to do?   **3 marks**

- Mobilise the surrounding bowels
- Suture the defect
- Technique/materials
- Consider defunctioning colostomy
- Continue division of adhesions to inspect the pelvic anatomy

Describe any measure you would take before closing the abdomen and technique for closure?   3 marks

- Uterus/tubes/ovaries

- Drains ? type

- Sutures – non-absorbable

- Further adhesions – prevention - Toilet/Dex

- Removal of suture

Postoperatively, how would you explain to the patient?   3 marks

- Appropriate language

- Adhesions

- Colostomy

- Nasogastric tube

- Cyst

- Drain

- Future prognosis

Global marks: 4 marks

TOTAL   **20 MARKS**

Emergency stations: example 2

CANDIDATE'S INSTRUCTIONS

You are the gynaecology registrar performing your own operating list. Your consultant is currently on the delivery suite performing a caesarean section. You are performing a caesarean section on a woman who has had two previous sections. There appear to be considerable difficulties with haemostasis. You have a suspicion of damaging the urinary bladder.

You are expected to describe to the examiner your management of this situation.

EXAMINER'S INSTRUCTIONS

The candidate has been given the following instructions: You are the gynaecology registrar performing your own operating list. Your consultant is currently on the delivery suite performing a caesarean section. You are performing a caesarean section on a woman who has had two previous sections. There appear to be considerable difficulties with haemostasis. You have a suspicion of damaging the urinary bladder.

Ask the candidate:

- What is your immediate action?

- Explain the principles behind your actions

- What would you say to this patient postoperatively and how would you manage her care?

MARKING SCHEME

Immediate actions: **4 marks**

- Call consultant – arrange transfusion and resuscitation – anaesthetic
- Confirm bladder perforation (inspection/Foley catheter/blue dye)
- Assess position of damage
- Decide if urological assistance required.

Principles of actions: haemostasis and suture: **6 marks**

- Check patient has prophylactic antibiotics
- Check for extension of tear
- Foley catheter (or suprapubic) (instruct staff to keep in for 7–10 days)
- Write full operation notes
- Redivac drain

Follow up action: **8 marks**

- Explanation to patient, preferably day one post operatively
- Explanation of any extenuating circumstances likely to have been discussed
- Need for large gauge catheter to stay in for 7–10 days (not permanent)
- Do not expect any long-term problems
- Future fertility
- Postoperative care
- Ensure staff understand need for continuous bladder

drainage for 10 days

- Catheter specimen of urine on day 2/3

- Consultant review before discharge (inform colleague of event)

- Ensure patient is followed up in gynaecological outpatient department by consultant

- Inform GP.

Global marks: **4 marks**

TOTAL   **20 MARKS**

Risk management stations

You will need a working knowledge of the principles of risk management. There is a very useful RCOG document on risk management (*Clinical Risk Management for Obstetricians and Gynaecologists.* Clinical Governance Advice No. 2), the latest version of which may be found on the College website at www.rcog.org.uk.

Risk management comprises three main areas:

- identification

- analysis

- control.

This can also be summarised as: 'What could go wrong?'; 'How did it go wrong?' and 'How can we stop it going wrong again?'.

It is important to understand how risk management works in practice: defined problems should prompt a clinical incident report. These are then collated into a database so that they can be analysed. The analysis should identify trends, either in clinical problems or individuals, which can then be addressed. Blame will not be apportioned. Serious incidents or trends can be analysed in particular detail, such as root cause analysis. This should produce a series of recommendations for reducing the risk in future.

Bouncers

PATHOLOGY

Hope it does not come up!

> **TOP TIP**
>
> Revise likely slides, especially cervical intraepithelial neoplasia (CIN) and dyskaryosis; ovarian pathology.

EXAMPLE TOPICS

- Dyskaryosis and cervical intraepithelial neoplasia.
- Ovarian tumour.

One candidate's experience of the Part 2 OSCE

STATION 1

A primiparous woman's labour is stuck at 8 cm for 6 hours and she has had oxytocin. A decision has been taken to perform a caesarean section. There was a long description of this woman's labour (about one side of A4 paper). It took me some time to read and this is part of your 15 minutes.

At the bottom of the sheet it said, 'Discuss with your consultant (the examiner) the reasons for caesarean section, consent, preoperative care, about the caesarean section, postoperative care, postoperative counselling and future management'.

I went through it all but with such a long list I did not mention one point. I was also asked about how this caesarean section would be different to an elective breech at term and what features would confirm cephalopelvic disproportion at caesarean section.

STATION 2

This was a counselling scenario with a fresh stillbirth scenario. There was a woman sobbing loudly. Again, there was a long description of what had happened to this woman. I was not given any specific instructions, so I just started to counsel her in a sympathetic way. After some time, the examiner brought the session to an end. I scored full marks. The examiner said this was because I did not do what everyone who had been on one course had done (pat the woman's arm and offer tissues) which he found annoying.

STATION 3

Husband of woman at Station 2, 6 weeks later. He was extremely aggressive, shouting and leaning over the desk towards me. Vasa praevia had been the cause of the stillbirth and some postmortem results were available. There was no guidance on what I should do. I therefore went through the postmortem results and did some general counselling and chatting, which revealed what had happened (his wife suffered antepartum haemorrhage, the theatre was busy and by the time a caesarean section could be performed, the fetal heart rate could not be heard). The man remained angry for the entire 15 minutes, despite my best attempts. Very intimidating.

STATION 4

I was given a referral letter from a GP regarding a 30-year-old woman with a history of vaginal discharge. All tests performed by the GP had been normal. I was the doctor seeing this woman in the gynaecology outpatient department. In taking a history, I discovered that the woman's life was affected significantly by this discharge and she thought that everyone could smell it.

I said I wanted to examine her. This prompted the examiner to give me the examination findings, all of which were normal. The discussion then continued. The patient was dissatisfied with all of my suggestions. She was quite difficult and told me she was unhappy with my management. I eventually brought the consultation to an end, as it was not going well but I did arrange a further follow up – there are marks for this as well as for giving a leaflet on the subject.

STATION 5

A pregnant woman at about 27 weeks of gestation. There was a sheet with a few clinical details about the woman. I was asked to manage this patient. She was unsure of her dates but knew the date of her last menstrual period. There was an obstetric wheel on the table and you were meant to pick it up and calculate her gestational age.

The woman was tearful. You had to take a history, which I did, including a social history. I asked questions such as: Who was looking after her other child? What were her work arrangements, and so on. I asked about the examination and was given the findings. It sounded like a urinary tract infection with irritable uterine contractions. I then went on to reassure the woman and explain management. She remained tearful. This made me suspicious, as I thought I had been very reassuring. I finally asked her if there was something else troubling her. At this point she looked at the examiner and he nodded at her. She then told me that her husband had just died (I nearly did too). I then started to talk more relevantly about depression, support from her GP and midwife, etc.

STATION 6

This was interpretation of results and outpatient management. This station was tricky as the examiner also played the patient and it was difficult to imagine a short, thin, Chinese man as a 'woman who is 100 kg with dry skin, etc'. I was shown some blood results: prolactin levels were raised and the woman had a hypothyroid picture. The 'woman' then asked questions about her condition, its treatment, her future fertility and the long-term outlook. I thought that it was not going smoothly but I just could not see what the examiner was wanting. I did not do well at this station and it was the only one I did not finish.

STATION 7

This station was preceded by a 15-minute preparation station. I found this time was easily adequate and it gave me a few moments to recover from the previous stations.

Information was provided about the patients on a labour ward, as well as the staff available, the location of the consultant (in clinic). The ten cases were:

- a woman who has had an eclamptic fit

- a multiparous woman at 3 cm dilated, contracting, with membranes intact and a transverse lie

- a woman with abdominal pain at 28 weeks of gestation

- a woman with a twin pregnancy who was in labour at 33 weeks; twin one is cephalic

- as woman awaiting elective caesarean section scheduled for that morning

- a woman in uncomplicated labour under midwifery care

- a woman who has had a spontaneous vaginal delivery awaiting suturing; she is not bleeding

- a woman who has had a fetal blood sample taken some hours ago and who should be about to deliver; no information about when she started pushing

- a woman who was a 'domino' booking, who should have delivered about 6 hours ago; there is meconium present

- an undiagnosed breech at term in early labour; she is a primipara at about 4 cm diltated.

I put the women into categories according to risk: high, medium and low. This, I think, worked well and followed advice from a course that I had attended. I gave fairly detailed information as to what I would do in each room. I called the consultant from clinic (you were meant to do this). Having sorted the board out, I was asked some questions by the examiner. He did say that I had managed to avoid most of his direct questions by giving lots of information on each room. He asked about magnesium sulphate (its role and doses) the delivery of twins, the role of epidurals and my opinion on breech delivery. He wanted to know what I would call the consultant for and why.

STATION 8

I had to discuss how to audit a protocol. I cannot recall the protocol subject. The principles were along the lines of any straightforward audit. The examiner asked me to outline the general principles of audit and how it is conducted. This was something that I had prepared for during my revision period. As a consequence, it was not difficult. We did not spend much time looking at the actual detail of the protocol. If you had ever conducted an audit, it was easy.

STATION 9

This was a viva station on diathermy. I found this fairly difficult and it was made more so because of the examiner's instructions: 'I have several questions. I am not allowed to prompt you at any time. I will ask you the question. When you have completed your answer please indicate this, so that we can go onto the next question'. So, you end up finishing your answer and thinking, 'Do I say I have finished or shall I try and think up some more?' You do not know the total number of questions. Examples of the questions included:

- 'You are the most senior doctor in theatre and you are performing a hysterectomy. The diathermy does not work. What do you do?'

- 'What are the risks of diathermy when performing a total abdominal hysterectomy?'

- 'Having completed the hysterectomy, you discover that the patient has a third-degree burn where the diathermy pad was. What do you do?'

The following questions have yes or no as the answer:

- 'Can you open the skin with monopolar diathermy?'

- 'Can you open the abdomen with monopolar diathermy?'

- 'Can you open the peritoneum with monopolar diathermy'

- 'At total abdominal hysterectomy, can you ligate the infundibulopelvic ligament with monopolar diathermy?'

STATION 10

This took the form of a critical appraisal of a WellBeing of Women leaflet on endometriosis. There was a 15-minute preparatory station preceding it. The leaflet had been photocopied but cunningly, the inside cover was not included, which lists the information on when the leaflet was written and by whom. This was a key point. This particular leaflet was quite long and the 15 minutes of preparation was barely enough. I was expected to pick up a lot of detail. There was not adequate time to finish reading the leaflet. I must have looked worried but the examiner reassured me that this was OK. There was a little discussion about the treatment of endometriosis.

This candidate took the OSCE examination in 2000 – and passed.

Index